IT STARTS WITH PALEO RECIPES

COOKING AND BAKING WITH BERRIES

ELIZABETH VINE

ELIZABETH VINE

ISBN-10: 1511962542
ISBN-13: 978-1511962544

CONTENTS

COOKING AND BAKING WITH:

STRAWBERRY

KNOWN AS THE "QUEEN OF FRUITS" IN ASIAN CULTURES, STRAWBERRIES HELP BOOST SHORT TERM MEMORY, EASE INFLAMMATION, PROMOTE BONE AND EYE HEALTH AND HAVE ANTI-AGING PROPERTIES.

BREAKFAST – GRANOLA

INGREDIENTS:
1 CUP WILD ORGANIC FRESH STRAWBERRIES
¼ CUP ALMONDS
¼ CUP CASHEWS
½ CUP HAZELNUTS
1 TBSP PUMPKIN SEEDS
1 TBSP COCONUT FLAKES
1 TBSP HONEY

DIRECTIONS:

IN A BLENDER OR FOOD PROCESSOR COMBINE ALMONDS, CASHEWS AND HAZELNUTS AND QUICKLY CHOP INTO SMALL PIECES, CAREFUL NOT TO OVER DO IT AND CREATE A SPREAD! YOU CAN ALSO USE A KNIFE TO BREAK INTO SMALL PIECES.
PUT INTO A BOWL; ADD THE PUMPKIN SEEDS AND COCONUT FLAKES.
WASH AND HULL THE STRAWBERRIES AND CUT INTO SMALL CITE SIZED SLICES. ADD TO THE BOWL.
POUR ½ CUP OF ALMOND MILK INTO THE BOWL AND DRIZZLE HONEY ON TOP.
SERVE & ENJOY!

SMOOTHIE

INGREDIENTS:
1 CUP ORGANIC WILD FRESH STRAWBERRIES
4-5 ICE CUBES
1 CUP ALMOND MILK
2 TBSP ALMOND BUTTER (SMOOTH)

DIRECTIONS:
COMBINE IN A BLENDER AND BLEND UNTIL SMOOTH.
SERVE&ENJOY!

SALAD

INGREDIENTS:
10 ORGANIC WILD FRESH STRAWBERRIES
3 CUPS MIXED GREENS
1 AVOCADO
½ CUP WALNUTS
2 TBSP COLD PRESSED OLIVE OIL
4 TSP RAW HONEY
1 TBSP APPLE CIDER VINEGAR
1 TSP FRESHLY SQUEEZED LEMON JUICE

DIRECTIONS:
WASH AND HULL THE STRAWBERRIES, THINLY
SLICE LENGTHWISE.
PEEL THE AVOCADO AND CUT INTO THIN
PIECES LENGTHWISE.
IN A SMALL BOWL OR MUG, COMBINE THE
LEMON JUICE, OLIVE OIL, HONEY AND
VINEGAR AND STIR TOGETHER.
WASH THE MIXED GREENS AND PLACE INTO A
SALAD BOWL.
ADD THE STRAWBERRIES, AVOCADO AND
WALNUTS, AND TOP WITH HONEY
VINAIGRETTE.
SERVE&ENJOY!

SYRUP

INGREDIENTS:
½ LB ORGANIC WILD STRAWBERRIES
½ CUP HONEY
1 TBSP VANILLA EXTRACT

DIRECTIONS:
WASH AND HULL THE STRAWBERRIES IN COLD
WATER.
IN A SAUCEPAN, HEAT THE STRAWBERRIES AND
HONEY OVER A LOW-MED TEMPERATURE. USE
A SPOON TO SMASH THE STRAWBERRIES.
BRING TO A BOIL AND SIMMER FOR 10-12
MINUTES WITHOUT COVERING.
ADD THE VANILLA AND STIR.
SERVE&ENJOY!
THIS IS GREAT POURED OVER ALMOND FOUR
WAFFLES!

CHUTNEY

INGREDIENTS:
1 LB ORGANIC WILD FRESH STRAWBERRIES
2/3 CUP RAW HONEY
3 TBSP APPLE CIDER VINEGAR
2 TBSP GINGER ROOT
1 SERRANO CHILLI PEPPER
1 TSP CAYENNE POWDER
1 TSP CINNAMON
½ TSP GREEN CARDAMOM POWDER
1 TSP CHILLI FLAKES
1 TSP SEA SALT

DIRECTIONS:
WASH AND HULL THE STRAWBERRIES AND
MINCE THE GINGER AND SERRANO PEPPER
IN A SAUCEPAN, BRING THE STRAWBERRIES,
HONEY AND APPLE CIDER VINEGAR TO BOIL
AND COOK FOR 10MIN.
ADD THE GINGER, SERRANO CHILLI PEPPER,
SALT AND CAYENNE POWDER, COOKING FOR
ANOTHER 10 MINUTES.
STIR IN THE CARDAMOM AND CINNAMON AND
LET COOL.
SERVE&ENJOY!
A GREAT APPETIZER WITH SOME PALEO
FLATBREAD OR PART OF A DESSERT,
GARNISHED OVER COCONUT ICE CREAM OR
PALEO CAKE!

SPREAD

INGREDIENTS:
4 LBS ORGANIC WILD FRESH STRAWBERRIES
8 TBSP CHIA SEEDS
¼ CUP RAW HONEY

DIRECTIONS:
WASH AND HULL THE STRAWBERRIES, SLICING
INTO SMALL PIECES.
HEAT THE STRAWBERRIES AND HONEY IN A
SAUCEPAN OVER MEDIUM HEAT,
SMASHING THE STRAWBERRIES WITH A HAND
HELD MASHER.
BRING TO A BOIL AND SIMMER FOR 7 MINUTES.
STIR IN CHIA SEEDS AND COOK FOR 1 MINUTE.
STIR WELL AND REMOVE FROM HEAT.
LET SIT FOR 10 MINUTES.
SERVE&ENJOY!

DESSERT – MOUSSE!

INGREDIENTS:
1 CUP ORGANIC WILD FRESH STRAWBERRIES
¾ TSP UNFLAVOURED GELATINE
¼ TSP VANILLA EXTRACT
1 RIPE AVOCADO
1 TBSP RAW HONEY
1 CUP FULL FAT COCONUT MILK

DIRECTIONS:
WASH AND HULL THE STRAWBERRIES.
IN A FOOD PROCESSOR, ADD THE AVOCADO
HONEY AND COCONUT MILK AND PROCESS
UNTIL SMOOTH.
ADD THE STRAWBERRIES, GELATINE AND
VANILLA AND PROCESS UNTIL EVERYTHING IS
MIXED WELL TOGETHER.
USING A MIXER, MIX ON HIGHEST SPEED FOR 4-
5 MINUTES UNTIL EVERYTHING IS LIGHT AND
FLUFFY.
PLACE IN THE FRIDGE FOR 4-5 HOURS.
SERVE&ENJOY!
DRINK – LEMONADE!

INGREDIENTS:
12 ORGANIC WILD FRESH STRAWBERRIES
1 CUP FRESHLY SQUEEZED LEMON JUICE
1 TBSP MAPLE OR AGAVE SYRUP
6 CUPS WATER

DIRECTIONS:
WASH AND HULL THE STRAWBERRIES, CUTTING
INTO QUARTERS.
ADD ALL THE INGREDIENTS INTO A BLENDER,
AND BLEND UNTIL SMOOTH.
SERVE WITH A FEW ICE CUBES OR CHILL IN THE
FRIDGE FOR 1-2 HOURS.
SERVE&ENJOY!

BLUEBERRY

FAMOUS FOR THEIR ANTIOXIDANT PROPERTIES, THIS BERRY HAS THE *HIGHEST* ANTIOXIDANT CAPACITY OF ALL FRESH FRUIT. PROMOTE URINARY TRACT HEALTH, BRAIN HEALTH, AID WITH HEART DISEASE AND GREAT FOR DIGESTION REDUCING CONSTIPATION.

BREAKFAST - PANCAKES

INGREDIENTS:
¾ CUP ORGANIC WILD BLUEBERRIES
3 EGGS
1 1/2 CUPS ALMOND FLOUR
1 CUP OF ALMOND MILK (OR WATER)
1 TSP SEA SALT
2 TBSP COCONUT OIL

DIRECTIONS:
MEASURE OUT FLOUR INTO A BIG BOWL THROUGH A SIFTER.
COMBINE EGGS AND MILK OR WATER (OR 1/2 OF EACH) AND MIX WELL.
SLOWLY MIX IN THE LIQUID MIXTURE TO THE FLOUR IN THE BIGGER BOWL. MAKE SURE THE MIXTURE DOES NOT BECOME TOO RUNNY.

ADD THE SALT AND FRESH BLUEBERRIES AND
MIX EVERYTHING TOGETHER.
HEAT A TBSP OF OIL IN A FRYING PAN ON LOW-
MED HEAT.
FILL A LADLE WITH PANCAKE BATTER AND
POUR INTO THE PAN WHEN THE OIL IS HOT,
COOK FOR 2-3 MINUTES AND THEN FLIP.
REPEAT UNTIL ALL THE BATTER IS USED.
DRIZZLE WITH MAPLE SYRUP OR HONEY!
SERVE&ENJOY!

SMOOTHIE

INGREDIENTS:
2 CUPS OF FROZEN WILD BLUEBERRIES
2 RIPE BANANAS
1 CUP ALMOND MILK
1 TBSP HONEY
1 TSP CHIA SEEDS

DIRECTIONS:
PLACE ALL INGREDIENTS INTO A BLENDER.
BLEND FOR A COUPLE MINUTES; ADD WATER
AS NEEDED FOR DESIRED CONSISTENCY.
SERVE&ENJOY!

SALAD - SPINACH

INGREDIENTS:
1 CUP WILD ORGANIC FRESH BLUEBERRIES
3 CUPS FRESH SPINACH SALAD
2 MEDIUM SIZED ORANGES
1/3 CUP PECANS
1 TBSP COLD PRESSED OLIVE OIL
1 TBSP SUGAR-FREE WHITE WINE VINEGAR
2 TBSP FRESHLY SQUEEZED ORANGE JUICE
1 TBSP MAPLE SYRUP

DIRECTIONS:
WASH THE BLUEBERRIES AND SPINACH LEAVES
AND PUT INTO A LARGE SALAD BOWL.
PEEL THE ORANGES AND CUT INTO BITE SIZED
CHUNKS, ADD TO SALAD BOWL.
IN A SMALL DISH OR BOWL, COMBINE THE
OLIVE OIL, VINEGAR, FRESHLY SQUEEZE
ORANGE JUICE AND MAPLE SYRUP AND STIR
WELL TOGETHER WITH A FORK.
POUR THE DRESSING OVER THE SALAD AND
MIX WELL.
TOP WITH PECANS.
SERVE&ENJOY!

GLAZE

INGREDIENTS:
¼ CUP WILD ORGANIC FROZEN BLUEBERRIES (THAWED)
1 ½ CUP RAW HONEY
½ TSP OF VANILLA EXTRACT
1 TSP FRESH LEMON JUICE
2 TBSP ALMOND MILK

DIRECTIONS:
USE A BLENDER OR FORK TO MASH ALL THE BLUEBERRIES TOGETHER.
REMOVE MOST OF THE SKINS, LEAVING A FEW IN THE BOWL.
ADD THE HONEY, VANILLA, LEMON JUICE AND ALMOND MILK WHISKING WELL TOGETHER.
SLOWLY POUR IN A BIT MORE ALMOND MILK TO ENSURE A SMOOTH CONSISTENCY.
TOP OVER COCONUT ICE CREAM, BREAKFAST PANCAKES OR BALSAMIC MARINATED PORK CHOPS!
SERVE&ENJOY!

SALSA

INGREDIENTS:
2 CUPS ORGANIC WILD BLUEBERRIES
1 CUP FRESHLY SLICED MANGO
¼ CUP FRESHLY SQUEEZED LEMON JUICE
3 TBSP CILANTRO
2 JALAPENO PEPPERS
1/3 CUP RED OR ORANGE BELL PEPPER
1 TSP SEA SALT

DIRECTIONS:
WASH ALL BLUEBERRIES, CILANTRO, JALAPENO
PEPPERS AND BELL PEPPER IN COLD WATER.
SLICE MANGO INTO SMALL SQUARES AND
SQUEEZE THE LEMON JUICE.
FINELY CHOP THE CILANTRO, PEPPERS AND
BELL PEPPER.
COMBINE ALL THE INGREDIENTS IN A BOWL,
POUR THE LEMON JUICE OVER TOP AND ADD
THE SALT.
SERVE&ENJOY!

GREAT FOR DIPPING SWEET POTATO CHIPS OR
ON TOP OF ROAST CHICKEN BREASTS!

SPREAD

INGREDIENTS:
2 CUPS WILD ORGANIC FRESH BLUEBERRIES
2 TSP FRESHLY SQUEEZED LEMON JUICE
2 TBSP HONEY
1 ½ TSP UNFLAVOURED ALL NATURAL
GELATINE
¾ CUP WATER

DIRECTIONS:
SOAK THE GELATINE IN A ¼ CUP OF COLD
WATER AND PUT ASIDE.
IN A SAUCEPAN OVER MEDIUM HEAT, BRING
THE BLUEBERRIES, LEMON JUICE AND HONEY
TO A BOIL AND SIMMER FOR 7-9 MINUTES,
STIRRING OFTEN.
ADD THE BLUEBERRIES TO THE GELATINE
MIXTURE AND STIR.
POUR INTO HOT, STERILIZED JARS AND SEAL
WELL.
SERVE&ENJOY!
GREAT OVER PALEO CREPES, FLAT BREADS OR
SPREAD OVER MUFFINS!

DESSERT – SORBET!
*YOU'LL NEED AN ICE CREAM MAKER

INGREDIENTS:
4 CUPS OF ORGANIC WILD FRESH BLUEBERRIES
2 TBSP FRESH GINGER
½ CUP MAPLE SYRUP
2 TSP LEMON JUICE
1 TSP SEA SALT

DIRECTIONS:
MINCE THE GINGER VERY FINE AND ADD TO A
BLENDER OR FOOD PROCESSOR.
ADD THE BLUEBERRIES AND BLENDER
TOGETHER UNTIL VERY SMOOTH.
ADD THE MAPLE SYRUP, LEMON JUICE AND
SALT AND BLEND AGAIN.
POUR THE MIXTURE THROUGH A STRAINER,
AND KEEP IN THE FRIDGE FOR 2-3 HOURS.
PUT THE SORBET MIXTURE INTO AN ICE CREAM
MAKER AND CHURN (BEST TO USE THE
DIRECTIONS FOR YOUR MACHINE!)
KEEP THE SORBET IN THE FREEZER FOR 3-4
HOURS PRIOR TO SERVING.
SERVE&ENJOY!

COCKTAIL – MOJITO!

INGREDIENTS (MAKES 1):
8 THAWED WILD ORGANIC BLUEBERRIES
2 TBSP FRESHLY SQUEEZED LIME JUICE
1 TBSP AGAVE SYRUP
8 FRESH MINT LEAVES
½ CUP RUM
1 CUP ICE
2 TBSP SUGAR-FREE CLUB SODA

DIRECTIONS:
ADD THE BLUEBERRIES, LIME JUICE, AGAVE
SYRUP AND MINT LEAVES INTO A COCKTAIL
SHAKER.
USE A WOODEN SPOON TO BASH THE MINT
INTO THE LIME JUICE AND AGAVE SYRUP AND
BREAK UP THE BLUEBERRIES.
ADD THE RUM AND STIR WELL.
PUT ICE CUBES INTO A GLASS AND POUR
MIXTURE OVER TOP.
TOP WITH CLUB SODA.
SERVE&ENJOY!

RASPBERRY

RICH IN VITAMINS C, B-COMPLEX GROUP, K, FOLIC ACID AND MANY MINERALS SUCH AS POTASSIUM AND IRON, RASPBERRIES HAVE MANY HEALTH BENEFITS AGAINST CANCER, AGING, INFLAMMATION AND NEURO-DEGENERATIVE DISEASES.

BREAKFAST - BREAKFAST BAR

INGREDIENTS:
1 ½ CUPS ORGANIC FROZEN RASPBERRIES
1 1/3 CUPS DRIED SHREDDED COCONUT FLAKES
1 1/3 CUPS WALNUTS
12 PITTED MEDJOOL DATES
½ TSP VANILLA
2 TBSP CHIA SEEDS
1 TSP CINNAMON
1 TSP SEA SALT

DIRECTIONS:
USING A FOOD PROCESSOR, MIX 1 CUP COCONUT FLAKES, 1 CUP WALNUTS, ½ TSP VANILLA, ½ TSP CINNAMON AND ½ TSP SEA SALT FOR 1 MINUTE.
ADD IN 8 PITTED MEDJOOL DATES.
LINE A BAKING SHEET WITH WAX PAPER AND SPREAD OUT THE MIXTURE EVENLY.
PUT IN THE FRIDGE FOR 1 HOUR TO FIRM.
USING A FOOD PROCESSOR OR MIXER, COMPLETELY BLEND 1 ½ CUPS OF FROZEN

THAWED RASPBERRIES WITH 4 DATES.
ADD IN 2 TABLESPOONS OF CHIA AND LEAVE
FOR 10-15 MINUTES UNTIL COMPLETELY
THICKENS INTO A JAM-LIKE MIXTURE.
REMOVE THE CRUMBLE LAYER FROM THE
FRIDGE, AND SPREAD THE RASPBERRY JAM
MIXTURE ON TOP.
IN A MAGIC BULLET OR FOOD PROCESSOR,
CRUMBLE TOGETHER 1/3 CUP COCONUT
FLAKES, ½ CUP WALNUTS, ½ TSP CINNAMON
AND ½ TSP OF SALT.
SPRINKLE ON TOP OF MIXTURE.
LEAVE IN THE FRIDGE FOR 1-2 HOURS TO FIRM.
SERVE&ENJOY!

SMOOTHIE

INGREDIENTS:
½ CUP ORGANIC FRESH RASPBERRIES
1 CUP SPINACH
½ CUP ALMOND MILK
1 TSP MAPLE SYRUP
1 BANANA
2-3 ICE CUBES

DIRECTIONS:
PUT ALL THE INGREDIENTS TOGETHER IN A
BLENDER UNTIL THOROUGHLY SMOOTH.
SERVE&ENJOY!

SALAD

INGREDIENTS:
1 ½ CUPS ORGANIC FRESH RASPBERRIES
5 CUPS ARUGULA & RADICCHIO SALAD
1 RIPE MANGO
1 AVOCADO
½ CUP RED ONION
¼ CUP HAZELNUTS
¼ CUP COLD PRESSED OLIVE OIL
¼ CUP RED WINE VINEGAR
1 GARLIC CLOVE
1 TSP SEA SALT
1 TSP PEPPER

DIRECTIONS:
PUT ½ CUP FRESH RASPBERRIES, ¼ CUP OLIVE OIL, ¼ CUP WINE VINEGAR, 1 MINCED GARLIC CLOVE, 1 TSP EACH SEA SALT AND PEPPER IN A BLENDER UNTIL SMOOTH TO MAKE A DRESSING.
WASH ARUGULA AND RADICCHIO SALAD LEAVES AND PLACE IN A BIG BOWL.
CUT THE MANGO AND AVOCADO INTO SMALL BITE SIZED QUARTERS AND ADD TO BOWL.
CHOP ½ CUP RED ONION AND ADD TO BOWL.
POUR THE SALAD DRESSING ON TOP AND MIX WELL.
TOP WITH 1 CUP FRESH RASPBERRIES AND ¼ CUP HAZELNUTS.
SERVE&ENJOY!

WHIPPED CREAM

INGREDIENTS:
½ CUP ORGANIC FRESH RASPBERRIES
1 TBSP RAW CACAO POWDER
½ TSP VANILLA
1 CAN FULL FAT COCONUT MILK
1 TSP RAW HONEY

DIRECTIONS:
KEEP THE CAN OF COCONUT MILK IN THE
FRIDGE FOR AT LEAST 6 HOURS (BEST TO DO IT
OVER NIGHT).
OPEN THE CAN OF COCONUT MILK AND POUR
OUT THE MILK, LEAVING THE SOLID COCONUT
CREAM.
PUT THE COCONUT CREAM INTO A COLD BOWL.
ADD THE FRESH RASPBERRIES, 1 TBSP RAW
CACAO POWDER, ½ TSP VANILLA AND 1 TSP
HONEY INTO THE BOWL.
USE A MIXER TO BLEND UNTIL THICKNESS OF
REGULAR WHIPPED CREAM.
SERVE&ENJOY!

THIS IS A *FANTASTIC* TOPPING FOR DESSERTS,
BREAKFAST WAFFLES/PANCAKES, OR SERVED
ON TOP OF A BOWL OF FRESH BERRIES.

CHUTNEY

INGREDIENTS:
1 CUP ORGANIC FROZEN RASPBERRIES
1 MEDIUM ONION
3 GARLIC CLOVES
1 CUP ALL NATURAL, NO SUGAR CHICKEN

BROTH
1 RED BELL PEPPER
1/3 CUP HONEY
1 GINGER ROOT
3 TBSP APPLE CIDER VINEGAR
1 CAN CHIPOTLE CHILLI IN ADOBO SAUCE
FRESH BUNDLE OF CILANTRO
1 TBSP AVOCADO OIL
SEA SALT
PEPPER

DIRECTIONS:
OVER MEDIUM TEMPERATURE, HEAT 1 TBSP
AVOCADO OIL IN A SAUCEPAN.
CHOP THE MEDIUM ONION AND ADD TO HOT
OIL, COOKING UNTIL ITS TRANSLUCENT (3-5
MIN).
MINCE GARLIC CLOVES AND ADD TO
SAUCEPAN, COOKING FOR ANOTHER 1-2
MINUTES.

ADD 1 CUP OF THE CHICKEN BROTH, ½
CHOPPED RED PEPPER, 1/3 CUP HONEY, 1 TBSP
MINCED GINGER ROOT, 3 TBSP CIDER VINEGAR
AND THE CAN OF CHIPOTLE CHILLI.
BRING TO A BOIL AND LET SIMMER FOR 2 ½
HOURS, STIRRING OFTEN.
ADD 1 CUP OF FROZEN, THAWED RASPBERRIES
AND COOK STIRRING FREQUENTLY FOR 15
MINUTES.
SET ASIDE AND LET COOL FOR 30 MINUTES.
CHOP A ¼ CUP OF FRESH CILANTRO AND ADD
TO SAUCEPAN ALONG WITH 1 TSP SEA SALT
AND PEPPER.
SERVE&ENJOY!

SERVE WITH MEATS, AS A SIDE DISH, OR A
CONDIMENT WITH PALEO WRAPS AND FLAT
BREADS!
REFRIGERATE AND USE A TSP – LASTS FOR
WEEKS!

SPREAD

INGREDIENTS:
2 ½ CUPS FRESH RASPBERRIES
1 TBSP FRESHLY SQUEEZED LEMON JUICE
1 TBSP RAW HONEY
1 TSP GELATINE

DIRECTIONS:
USE A MASHER TO CRUSH THE RASPBERRIES
AND PUT THROUGH A STRAINER, LEAVING
LITTLE LIQUID.
PUT INTO A BOWL AND ADD THE LEMON JUICE,
RAW HONEY AND A 1 TSP OF GELATINE MIXING
WELL TOGETHER.
SET ASIDE FOR 30-45 MINUTES.
FREEZE AND USE AS NEEDED.
SERVE&ENJOY!

DESSERT

INGREDIENTS:
¾ CUP ORGANIC FRESH RASPBERRIES
2 CUPS ALMOND FLOUR
1 ORGANIC ORANGE
2/3 CUP RAW HONEY
1 TSP BAKING POWDER
½ TSP BAKING SODA
½ TSP GROUND CARDAMOM
½ TSP GROUND GINGER POWDER
½ TSP HIMALAYAN PINK SEA SALT
3 ORGANIC, FREE RANGE LOCAL EGGS
¼ CUP COLD PRESSED OLIVE OIL
½ CUP RAW PISTACHIOS

DIRECTIONS:
PREHEAT THE OVEN TO 325F.
IN A MIXING BOWL, ADD THE ALMOND FLOUR,
BAKING POWDER, BAKING SODA, CARDAMOM,
GINGER AND SEA SALT.
IN A SEPARATE BOWL, BEAT THE EGGS AND
ADD THE HONEY, OLIVE OIL AND ZEST OF
ORANGE INTO IT.
USE A WHISK TO MIX THE WET BOWL VERY
WET.
POUR THE WET BOWL INTO THE DRY, STIRRING
UNTIL NO MORE CLUMPS REMAIN.
ADD IN WASHED, FRESH RASPBERRIES AND STIR
WITH A WOODEN SPOON.
GREASE A PAN (PREF 9") WITH OLIVE OIL, AND
A BIT OF ALMOND FLOUR.

POUR THE MIXTURE INTO THE PAN AND
PREAD EVENLY.
BAKE FOR 45-50 MINUTES UNTIL A TOOTHPICK
COMES OUT WITH NO WET DOUGH WHEN
INSERTED.
COOL THE CAKE TO A ROOM TEMPERATURE.
SQUEEZE JUICE OF ½ THE ORANGE AND ADD 1
TSP OF HONEY INTO IT.
ADD THE PISTACHIOS INTO THE JUICE AND
COAT.
SPREAD OVER THE CAKE WHEN COOLED.
SERVE&ENJOY!

COCKTAIL

INGREDIENTS:

**USE THE SPREAD RECIPE FOR THIS COCKTAIL!
1 TBSP FRESHLY SQUEEZED LEMON JUICE
1 OZ ALL NATURAL CRANBERRY JUICE
1 OZ MAPLE SYRUP
2 OZ VODKA
1 TBSP RASPBERRY SPREAD
3-4 ICE CUBES
1 CAN OF NO SUGAR CLUB SODA
A FRESH RASPBERRY FOR GARNISH

DIRECTIONS:
ADD THE LEMON JUICE, CRANBERRY JUICE,
MAPLE SYRUP, VODKA, JAM AND ICE IN A
COCKTAIL SHAKER AND SHAKE.
ADD 2 ICE CUBES TO A COCKTAIL GLASS AND
POUR COCKTAIL MIXTURE OUT OF SHAKER ON
TOP.
ADD A SPLASH OF CLUB SODA AND GARNISH
WITH 1-3 FRESH RASPBERRIES.
SERVE&ENJOY!

BLACKBERRY

AS THE BERRY WITH THE HIGHEST FIBRE CONTENT, BLACKBERRIES ARE HIGHLY BENEFICIAL IN AIDING SKIN HEALTH, WOMEN'S HEALTH CANCER PREVENTION AND DIGESTIVE TRACT HEALTH.

BREAKFAST

INGREDIENTS:
½ CUP ORGANIC FRESH BLACKBERRIES
1 ¾ CUPS ALMOND FLOUR
3 TBSP COCONUT FLOUR
¼ CUP RAW HONEY
1 EGG
¼ CUP ALMOND MILK
3 TBSP COCONUT OIL
1 TSP BAKING SODA
1 TSP SEA SALT

DIRECTIONS:
PREHEAT OVEN TO 350F.
PUT THE ALMOND FLOUR, COCONUT FLOUR, SALT AND BAKING SODA INTO A BOWL.
IN A SEPARATE BOWL, COMBINE THE HONEY, EGG, ALMOND MILK AND MELTED COCONUT OIL.
MIX IN THE WET INGREDIENTS INTO THE DRY INGREDIENTS.
WASH THE BLACKBERRIES AND FOLD INTO THE

DOUGH WITH A WOODEN SPOON.
USING A TABLESPOON, SCOOP OUT A FULL
SPOONFUL AND SHAPE INTO A SCONE
TRIANGLE PLACING ONTO A GREASED BAKING
SHEET.
REPEAT UNTIL ALL DOUGH IS USED UP.
BAKE FOR 20 MINUTES UNTIL TURN GOLDEN
BROWN.
SERVE&ENJOY!

SMOOTHIE

INGREDIENTS:
½ CUP ORGANIC FROZEN BLACKBERRIES
½ CUP ORGANIC FROZEN STRAWBERRIES
1 CUP KALE
1 TBSP ALMOND BUTTER
2 TSP CHIA SEEDS
1 TSP HEMP SEEDS
¾ CUP ALMOND MILK
3-4 ICE CUBES

DIRECTIONS:
COMBINE ALL INGREDIENTS INTO A BLENDER
AND MIX UNTIL SMOOTH.
SERVE&ENJOY!

SALAD

INGREDIENTS:
1 CUP ORGANIC FRESH BLACKBERRIES
4 SLICES OF BACON
4 CUPS FRESH BABY SPINACH
1/3 CUP ALMONDS
4 ORGANIC GRAPE TOMATOES
½ CUP COLD PRESSED OLIVE OIL
¼ CUP WHITE BALSAMIC VINEGAR
1 GARLIC CLOVE
1 TSP MUSTARD

1 TSP SEAL SALT
1 TSP BLACK PEPPER

DIRECTIONS:
IN A MEDIUM SAUCEPAN, OVER MED-HIGH
TEMPERATURE, COOK BACON SLICES UNTIL
CRISPY.
PUT ASIDE ON A PLATE LINED WITH PAPER
TOWEL.
IN A BLENDER COMBINE 1 CUP WASHED
BLACKBERRIES, MINCED GARLIC CLOVE,
MUSTARD, AND WHITE BALSAMIC VINEGAR.
SLOWLY ADD IN THE OLIVE OIL AND BLEND
UNTIL EVERYTHING IS THOROUGHLY MIXED.
ADD SALT AND PEPPER AND SET VINAIGRETTE
ASIDE.
WASH THE SPINACH LEAVES AND PUT INTO A
BOWL.
CRUMBLE THE CRISPY BACON AND PUT INTO
THE BOWL.
WASH AND SLICE THE GRAPE TOMATOES, ADD
TO THE BOWL.
ADD THE ALMONDS AND FRESH BLACKBERRIES
TO THE BOWL.
ADD THE SALAD DRESSING AND MIX
THOROUGHLY.
SERVE&ENJOY!

GLAZE – JALAPENO BLACKBERRY

INGREDIENTS:
½ CUP ORGANIC FRESH BLACKBERRIES
1 TBSP UNPASTEURIZED BUTTER
2 JALAPENOS
1 GARLIC CLOVES
1 CUP ORGANIC, NO SULPHITE, RED WINE
½ TSP TAPIOCA FLOUR

DIRECTIONS:
BROIL THE JALAPENOS IN THE OVEN FOR 3-5
MINUTES ON EACH SIDE UNTIL ROASTED (BUT
NOT BURNT!).
REMOVE AND SET ASIDE, CHOPPING FINELY
WHEN COOLED.
PUT THE BLACKBERRIES THROUGH A FOOD
PROCESSOR.
IN A SAUCEPAN OVER MED-HIGH HEAT, MELT
THE BUTTER.
ADD THE ROASTED JALAPENOS AND MINCED
GARLIC CLOVE AND COOK FOR 3-4 MINUTES.
ADD THE PROCESSED BLACKBERRIES AND CUP
OF RED WINE.
BRING TO A BOIL AND SIMMER FOR 20-25
MINUTES.
ADD THE TAPIOCA FLOUR AND A SPLASH MORE
RED WINE AND COOK FOR ANOTHER 5
MINUTES.
POUR OVER RIBS, PORK CHOPS OR SLICE OF
HAM.
SERVE&ENJOY!

SALSA

INGREDIENTS:
2 CUPS ORGANIC FRESH BLACKBERRIES
½ RED ONION
½ JALAPENO
½ CUP CHOPPED FRESH CILANTRO
1 LIME
1 TBSP SEA SALT
1 TBSP PEPPER

DIRECTIONS:
FINELY CHOP THE RED ONION, JALAPENO AND
CILANTRO AND PUT INTO A BOWL.
WASH THE BLACKBERRIES AND ADD TO BOWL.
SQUEEZE THE JUICE OF THE LIME AND ADD
SALT AND PEPPER.
MIX ALTOGETHER WELL.
SERVE&ENJOY!
GREAT AS A DIPPING SAUCE FOR
SWEETPOTATO OR CARROT CHIPS! ALSO GREAT
ON TURKEY PATTIES!

SPREAD

INGREDIENTS:
2 ½ CUPS ORGANIC FROZEN BLACKBERRIES
4 CUPS FRESH BASIL LEAVES
½ CUP RAW HONEY
¼ CUP FRESHLY SQUEEZED ORANGE JUICE
4 TBSP FRESHLY SQUEEZED LEMON

DIRECTIONS:
THAW THE BLACKBERRIES AND ALONG WITH
THE JUICE, PUT INTO A SAUCEPAN AND MASH
WELL.
COMBINE THE BASIL, HONEY, ORANGE AND
LEMON JUICE IN A FOOD PROCESSOR AND
BLEND UNTIL THOROUGHLY SMOOTH.
PUT INTO THE SAUCEPAN AND HEAT OVER
MEDIUM TEMPERATURE, BRINGING TO A BOIL.
SIMMER, STIRRING OCCASIONALLY, FOR 25-30
MINUTES.
ALLOW TO COOL AND THICKEN FOR 1-2 HOURS,
REFRIGERATING.
SERVE&ENJOY!

DESSERT

INGREDIENTS:
1 ½ CUPS ORGANIC FROZEN BLACKBERRIES
2 TBSP MAPLE SYRUP
1 CUP ALMOND MILK
3 TBSP CACAO POWDER
1 TSP RAW HONEY OR AGAVE SYRUP
4 CUPS COCONUT ICE CREAM

DIRECTIONS:
IN A MEDIUM SAUCEPAN, HEAT THE
BLACKBERRIES AND MAPLE SYRUP OVER MED-
HIGH TEMP FOR 5-6 MINUTES.
PUT THE BERRIES + JUICES INTO A BLENDER,
WITH 4 CUPS COCONUT ICE CREAM (HOME
MADE OR STORE BOUGHT, SUGAR FREE!),
ALMOND MILK AND CACAO POWDER AND
BLEND UNTIL COMPLETELY SMOOTH.
POUR INTO DESSERT CUPS AND OPTION TO
FREEZE FIRST.
SERVE&ENJOY!

COCKTAIL

INGREDIENTS:
5 ORGANIC FRESH BLACKBERRIES
6 MINT LEAVES
2 OZ TEQUILA
1 OZ JUICE OF LIME
1 OZ HONEY SYRUP (1/2 HONEY, ½ WATER)
5-6 ICE CUBES

DIRECTIONS:
MASH THE MINT LEAVES AND BLACKBERRIES
IN A COCKTAIL SHAKER.
ADD THE TEQUILA, LIME JUICE, HONEY SYRUP
AND ICE CUBES AND SHAKE.
FILL A GLASS WITH ICE CUBES AND POUR OUT
OF COCKTAIL SHAKER ON TOP OF ICE.
GARNISH WITH FRESH BLACKBERRIES!
SERVE&ENJOY!

GOOSEBERRY

RICH IN NUTRIENTS, GOOSEBERRIES IMPROVE EYE VISION, SKIN AND HAIR HEALTH, AS WELL AS PROMOTE NERVOUS SYSTEM, MEMORY AND BRAIN HEALTH.

SAUCE

INGREDIENTS:
1 CUP OR GOOSEBERRIES
2 TBSP RAW HONEY
1 MEDIUM ONION

DIRECTIONS:
USING SCISSORS SNIP EACH END OF THE GOOSEBERRIES AND WASH THEM THOROUGHLY.
PUT INTO A SAUCEPAN WITH 1/3 CUP OF WATER OVER MEDIUM HEAT AND ADD HONEY AND FINELY CHOPPED MEDIUM ONION.
COOK FOR 10-15 MINUTES UNTIL THE BERRIES ARE SOFT.
POUR OVER SALMON OR PORK CHOPS AS A SAUCE.
SERVE&ENJOY!

DESSERT – GOOSEBERRY CUPS!

INGREDIENTS:
1 CUP FRESH GOOSEBERRIES
1/3 CUP COCONUT MILK
1 EGG
3 TBSP MAPLE SYRUP
2 TBSP KOMBUCHA

DIRECTIONS:
PREHEAT THE OVEN TO 350F.
USING SCISSOR SNIP EACH END OF THE
GOOSEBERRIES AND RINSE WITH COLD WATER.
PUT THEM WHOLE INTO SILICONE CUPCAKE
CASINGS.
SEPARATE THE WHOLE CREAM OUT OF THE
CAN OF COCONUT MILK AND MEASURE OUT 1/3
CUP.
WHISK THE COCONUT CREAM WITH 1 EGG,
MAPLE SYRUP AND KOMBUCHA TOGETHER
AND POUR OVER THE BERRIES.
BAKE FOR 15-18 MINUTES AND REMOVE FROM
OVEN.
SERVE&ENJOY!

HUCKLEBERRY

BEST KNOWN TO CONTAIN HIGH LEVELS OF
VITAMIN B AND C, HUCKLEBERRIES ARE
ESSENTIAL IN IMPROVING METABOLISM AND
ENHANCING CELL GROWTH. ALSO KNOWN TO
ENHANCE FUNCTIONS OF PANCREAS AND AID
IN DIGESTION, AS WELL AS HELP TO PREVENT
PANCREATIC CANCER.

BREAKFAST - MUFFINS

INGREDIENTS:
1/3 CUP FRESH HUCKLEBERRIES
1 CUP ALMOND FLOUR
¼ TSP BAKING SODA
2 TBSP RAW HONEY
½ CUP FULL FAT COCONUT MILK
1 EGG
1 TSP SEA SALT
   2 TSP COCONUT OIL

DIRECTIONS:
PREHEAT THE OVEN TO 350F.
IN A BOWL, MIX IN THE ALMOND FLOUR,
BAKING SODA AND SALT.
IN A SEPARATE BOWL, MIX IN THE COCONUT
MILK, EGG, HONEY AND MELTED COCONUT
OIL.
WHISK TOGETHER THE WET BOWL AND
SLOWLY FOLD INTO THE DRY MIXTURE.

WASH THE HUCKLEBERRIES AND ADD INTO
THE BATTER.
BAKE IN A GREASED MUFFIN TRAY 20-25
MINUTES UNTIL GOLDEN BROWN.
SERVE&ENJOY!

SMOOTHIE

INGREDIENTS:
½ CUP ORGANIC WILD HUCKLEBERRIES
½ CUP ORGANIC FRESH CHERRIES
1 BANANA
½ ORANGE
1 CUP COCONUT WATER

DIRECTIONS:
PUT ALL INGREDIENTS IN A BLENDER UNTIL
SMOOTH.
SERVE&ENJOY!

BOYSENBERRY

BOYSENBERRIES HAVE A POWERFUL, UNIQUE ANTIOXIDANT TO THIS BERRY THAT IS EXTREMELY IMPORTANT TO BRAIN HEALTH AND IS MOST WELL KNOWN FOR BRAIN FUNCTION AND PREVENTION OF MEMORY LOSS AND DISEASE.

DESSERT - SORBET

INGREDIENTS:
4 CUPS FRESH LOCAL BOYSENBERRIES
¼ CUP MAPLE SYRUP
¼ CUP WATER
HANDFUL OF VERBENA

DIRECTIONS:
IN A SAUCEPAN OVER LOW HEAT, BRING THE MAPLE SYRUP AND WATER TO A BOIL.
ADD THE VERBENA AND SIMMER FOR 3-5 MINUTES.
PUT ASIDE AND PUT IN THE FRIDGE OVERNIGHT.
PLACE THE BOYSENBERRIES INTO A FOOD PROCESSOR AND BLEND UNTIL SMOOTH.

ALSO PLACE IN THE FRIDGE OVERNIGHT.
THE NEXT DAY MIX THE TWO TOGETHER AND
PUT THROUGH YOUR ICE CREAM MAKER,
FOLLOWING INSTRUCTIONS AS PER YOUR
SPECIFIC MACHINE.
FREEZE FOR 5-6 HOURS.
SERVE&ENJOY!

DESSERT - BOYSENBERRY PIE

INGREDIENTS:
2 CUPS ORGANIC LOCAL BOYSENBERRIES
2 CUPS ALMOND FLOUR
¼ + 4 TSP CUP TAPIOCA FLOUR
1 TSP SEA SALT
¼ TSP BAKING SODA
½ CUP PURE MAPLE SYRUP
1 TBSP VANILLA
½ CUP COCONUT OIL
½ CUP WATER
1 TSP FRESHLY SQUEEZED LEMON JUICE

DIRECTIONS:
PREHEAT OVEN TO 350F.
IN A LARGE BOWL, COMBINE THE ALMOND
FLOUR, TAPIOCA FLOWER, SALT AND BAKING
SODA.
IN ANOTHER BOWL, WHISK MELTED COCONUT
OIL, MAPLE SYRUP AND VILLA.
SLOWLY MIX IN THE WET MIXTURE INTO THE
DRY.
POUR THE MIXTURE AND PRESS IN WELL TO A
10" PIE PAN.
BAKE FOR 15 MINUTES UNTIL STARTS TO TURN
A GOLDEN COLOUR.
LET IT COOL FOR 10 MINUTES AND REMOVE
THE SHELL.
IN A SAUCEPAN, BRING THE BOYSENBERRIES, ¼
CUP OF MAPLE SYRUP, 4 TSP TAPIOCA FLOUR
AND ½ CUP WATER TO A BOIL.
MASH EVERYTHING WELL TOGETHER AND STIR
UNTIL STARTS TO THICKEN.
REMOVING FROM THE STOVE, ADD 1 TBSP
MELTED COCONUT OIL, 1 TSP FRESHLY
SQUEEZED LEMON JUICE AND STIR.
PLACE INTO THE PIE SHELL AND PUT IN THE
FRIDGE FOR 1-2 HOURS.
SERVE&ENJOY!

**WATERMELON

ALTHOUGH THIS ONE DOES NOT TECHNICALLY FALL INTO THE "BERRY" SECTION – IT IS A SUMMER *FAVOURITE* GO TO FRUIT WITH MANY HEALTH BENEFITS. MOST WELL KNOWN FOR ITS ANTI-INFLAMMATORY SUPPORT, THIS ONE IS KEY FOR CARDIOVASCULAR HEALTH, CONTAINING MANY AMINO ACIDS THAT HELP IN KIDNEY FUNCTION.

SALAD

INGREDIENTS:
6 CUPS MIXED GREENS
2 CUPS WATERMELON CHUNKS
2 AVOCADOS
HANDFUL OF FRESH BASIL
3 TBSP BALSAMIC VINEGAR
2 TBSP COLD PRESSED OLIVE OIL
2 LIMES
1 TBSP RAW LOCAL HONEY

DIRECTIONS:
SQUEEZE JUICE OF LIMES AND WHISK TOGETHER WITH VINEGAR, OLIVE OIL AND HONEY.
CUT THE AVOCADOS AND WATERMELON INTO BITE SIZED CHUNKS.
WASH THE GREENS AND PUT INTO A BOWL.

ADD THE WATERMELON, AVOCADOS AND
FRESH BASIL.
DRIZZLE WITH SALAD DRESSING AND MIX
WELL TOGETHER.
SERVE&ENJOY!

DESSERT - WHOLE WATERMELON COCONUT
CAKE

INGREDIENTS:
1 LARGE SEEDLESS LOCAL WATERMELON
2 CUPS COCONUT MEAT
2 TBSP RAW HONEY
1 TSP VANILLA
2 TBSP FRESHLY SQUEEZED LEMON JUICE
2 TBSP COCONUT OIL
½ CUP ALMONDS
½ CUP BLUEBERRIES
1 KIWI
1 TSP SEA SALT

DIRECTIONS:
IN A BLENDER, MIX THE COCONUT MEAT,
HONEY, LEMON JUICE, VANILLA, MELTED
COCONUT OIL AND SALT UNTIL SMOOTH.
PUT INTO THE FRIDGE AND COOL FOR 20-30
MINUTES.
USING A SHARP KNIFE CUT THE CORE OFF THE
WATERMELON, LEAVING IT WHOLE.

TAKE THE FROSTING OUT OF THE FRIDGE AND COVER THE TOP AND SIDES OF THE WATERMELON WITH THE FILLING.
SLICE THE KIWI INTO THIN SLICES AND LAYER ON THE TOP.
POUR THE ½ CUP BLUEBERRIES IN THE CENTER OF THE KIWI SLICES.
PLACE COCONUT SHREDS AND ALMONDS ALONG THE SIDES.
KEEP IN THE FRIDGE UNTIL READY TO EAT.
SERVE&ENJOY!

THANK YOU!!

FOR BUYING OUR
IT STARTS WITH PALEO RECIPES

WE HOPE YOU ENJOYED MAKING AND EATING
THE RECIPES AS MUCH AS WE ENJOYED
PUTTING THEM TOGETHER (AND TESTING
THEM! YUMM!).

NOW THAT YOU'VE SEEN HOW DELICIOUS
EATING PALEO IS AND YOU'RE READY TO
MAKE IT A LIFESTYLE – WE'VE PUT TOGETHER
A FREE THANK YOU GIFT FOR YOU.

IF WE CAN TAKE A SECOND AND ASK YOU FOR
A SMALL FAVOUR??

IF YOU ENJOYED THIS BOOK PLEASE LET US AN
HONEST REVIEW ON AMAZON.COM.
REVIEWS ARE SO IMPORTANT FOR
INDEPENDENT AUTHORS LIKE US AND IT
WOULD MEAN A HUGE AMOUNT IF YOU TOOK
THE 2 MINUTES TO WRITE ONE.

TO DOWNLOAD YOUR FREE GIFT PLEASE GO
TO:
HTTP://WWW.PALEOWIRED.COM/FREE-PALEO-
INTRODUCTION/

www.ingramcontent.com/pod-product-compliance
Lightning Source LLC
Chambersburg PA
CBHW070828290526
45795CB00002B/867